# better together*

*This book is best read together, grownup and kid.

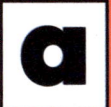 **akidsco.com**

a
kids
book
about

# a kids book about

# YOGA

by Megan Snider

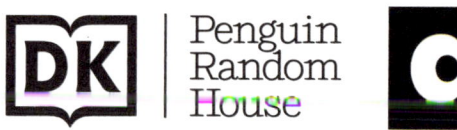

**A Kids Co.**
**Editor** Emma Wolf
**Designer** Rick DeLucco
**Creative Director** Rick DeLucco
**Studio Manager** Kenya Feldes
**Sales Director** Melanie Wilkins
**Head of Books** Jennifer Goldstein
**CEO and Founder** Jelani Memory

**DK**
**Senior Production Editor** Jennifer Murray
**Senior Production Controller** Louise Minihane
**Senior Acquisitions Editor** Katy Flint
**Acquisitions Project Editor** Sara Forster
**Managing Art Editor** Vicky Short
**Managing Director, Licensing** Mark Searle

First American edition, 2025
Published in the United States by DK Publishing, 1745 Broadway, 20th Floor,
New York, NY 10019

First published in Great Britain in 2025 by
Dorling Kindersley Limited, 20 Vauxhall Bridge Road, London SW1V 2SA
A Penguin Random House Company

The authorised representative in the EEA is
Dorling Kindersley Verlag GmbH. Arnulfstr. 124, 80636 Munich, Germany

A catalog record for this book is available from the Library of Congress.
A CIP catalogue record for this book is available from the British Library.
ISBN: 978-0-2417-4310-2

DK books are available at special discounts when purchased in bulk for sales
promotions, premiums, fund-raising, or education use. For details, contact:
DK Publishing Special Markets, 1745 Broadway, 20th Floor, New York, NY 10019
SpecialSales@dk.com

Printed and bound in China
www.dk.com
akidsco.com

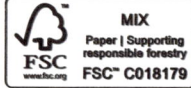

This book was made with Forest
Stewardship Council™ certified
paper – one small step in DK's
commitment to a sustainable future.
Learn more at www.dk.com/uk/
information/sustainability

For all of the kids who have ever felt unseen and unheard when being their truest selves. It was never your fault.

And for all those who helped me write this book: Andrew, Jadwin, Jethro, Fenix, Taryn, Kelly S., Pat, Elizabeth, and all my yoga and life teachers past, present, and future.

# Intro
## for grownups

Yoga is an often misunderstood topic in the global North. In our efforts to make yoga palatable, acceptable, and accessible for large audiences, we have lost a deeper connection to a rich tradition. Yoga is so much more than an exercise class and putting your body into postures.

Yoga is a vehicle for returning to our truest selves. And with yoga, we have support to raise connected, aware humans, teaching kids how to value and honor who they are with courage. Our world today can seem to be full of violence, hurt, and shame, and yoga helps us navigate through those experiences and learn from them. Yoga connects us to ourselves, our friends and families, and Earth—the things that really matter in life.

What would your childhood have been like if you were given the space and support to become your truest self? Yoga helps us do that, and that's why I teach yoga to kids.

# Rub your hands together.

Sit up nice and tall, reaching your spine and the crown of your head to the sky, and root your hips down into the earth.

Inhale to bring your
arms up over your head...

# and exhale, "Ahhh

hhhhhhhhhhhhhhh,"

to bring your hands down to your heart.

And do that one more time (I'll wait).

Now, just shake it out.

Shake your head, your shoulders, your ear lobes, your knees—shake it all out, and keep shaking...

and FREEZE!

Close your eyes,

breathe,

open them again,

and let's begin.

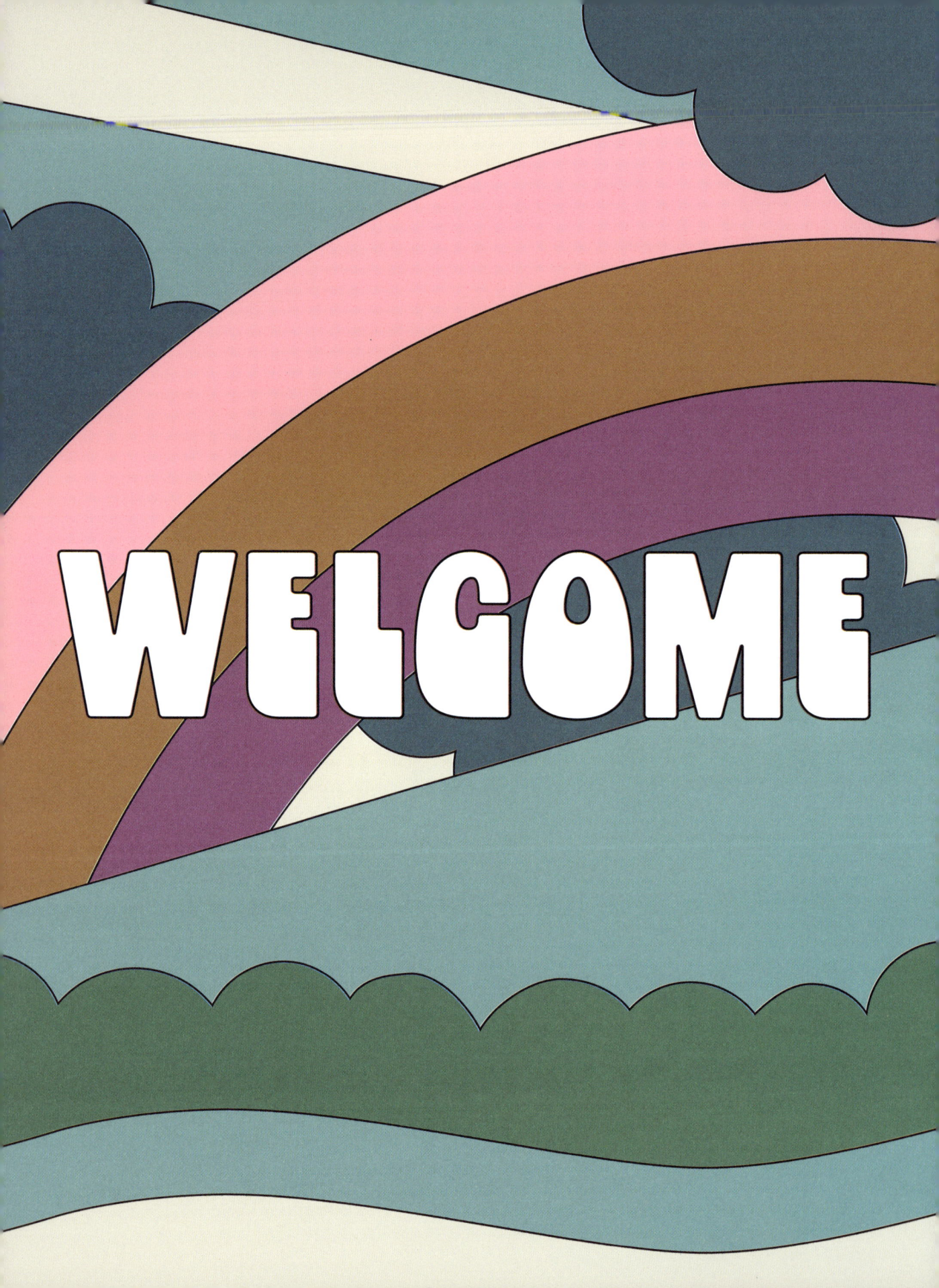

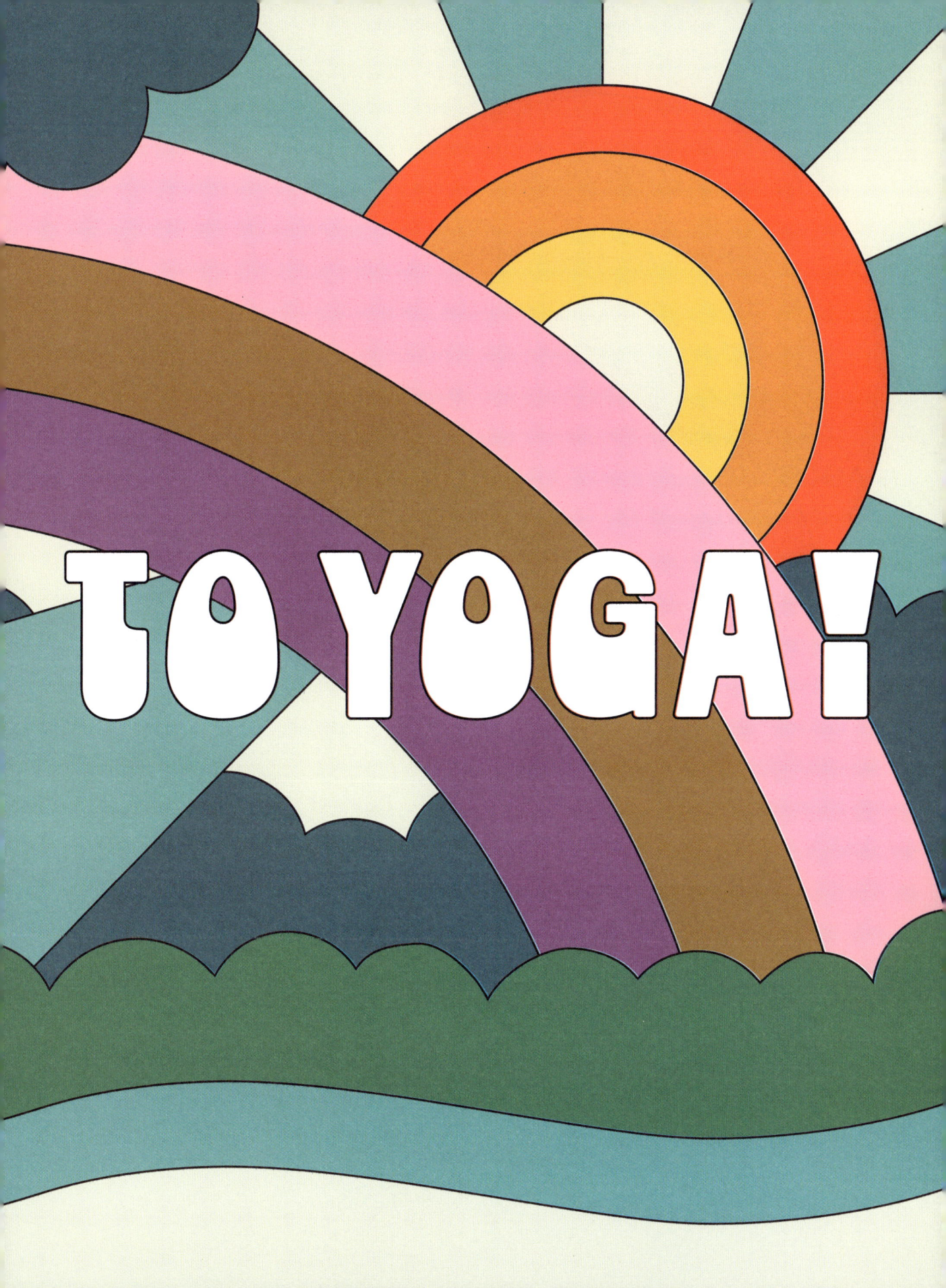

The word yoga means
to "join together."

It's like a hug you give to someone.

In that hug, you and that
person have connected.

"Yoga" comes from a Sanskrit verb meaning "joining together."

But it was originally used to describe a state or feeling:

peaceful and connected.

Later on, yoga became an activity to do in order to access that **peaceful state.**

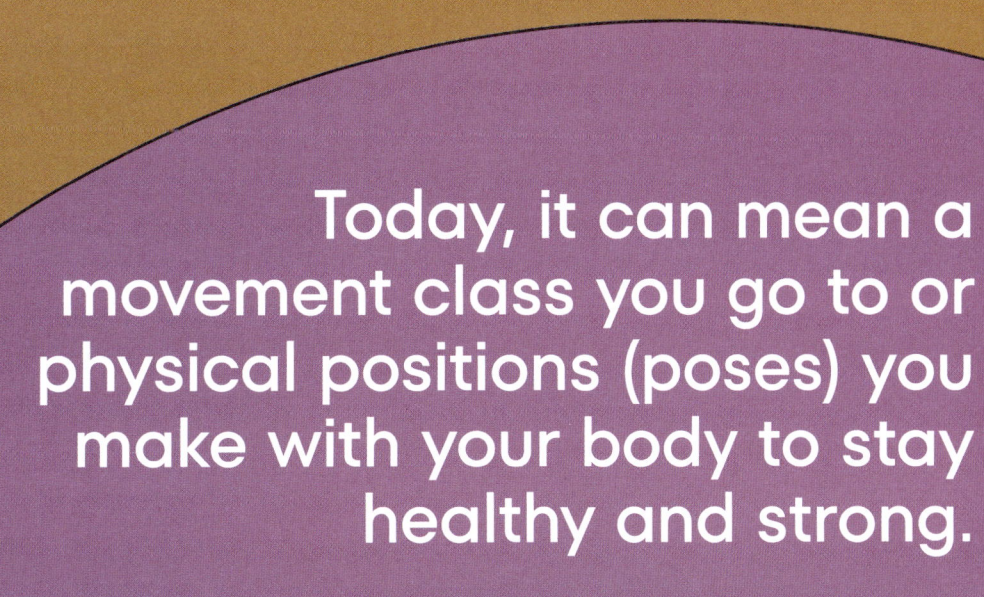

Today, it can mean a movement class you go to or physical positions (poses) you make with your body to stay healthy and strong.

Basically.............................................

the word "yoga" means many things.

Today, for me, yoga is how
I join together things that
were never meant to be apart:

me and nature,

me and my dad,

my mind
and my body,

and me and the
younger version
of myself who still
lives within me.

Yoga has been around
for a LONG time.

And it's different depending
on a person's age, what stage
of life they're in, and where
they live in the world.

Yoga changes with you. Like a good
friend, it grows alongside you.

We honor this good friend by remembering where the **tradition** of yoga comes from, in what we now call Southeast Asia, and in particular, India.

# Yoga is a practice and a philosophy.

I can practice *frog pose*, and I can use yoga as a way to see the world.

# Yoga is a way of thinking and solving problems.

When I know my mind and body better, I can also better understand my emotions and experiences.

If a yoga pose is like
a drop of water...

yoga itself is like

the whole ocean.

# Yoga reminds me how to be my truest self.

Like when I know I should
be truthful, even when it's hard.

Or when I need to apologize to
someone for hurting them.

If I can be my truest self, I can be a
better friend, mom, family member,
community member, and teacher.

Yoga also teaches me about my

# CONNECTION THINGS, INCLU AND MOTHER

# TO ALL LIVING DING MYSELF EARTH.

Yoga helps me focus
on myself and my body.

To connect with my breath, and how I'm feeling.

Yoga is about noticing
what is happening:

Oh, my knee hurts!

Wow, my mind is moving so fast.

My breathing is happening quickly.

Ugh, I feel sad today.

I feel like I don't belong.

I feel at peace.

In this way, I develop an awareness of my body and my mind.

When I'm doing yoga with my family,
I connect with them through...

touch,

eye contact,

creating new ways to move,

and listening.

We play together, choosing
to move and be present
with one another.

As a result of that,
we become more

# OPEN TO CURIOSITY AND JOY.

I learn so much from my kids. They allow me to connect with my own inner child.

In this state, I feel like the most free, most natural version of myself.

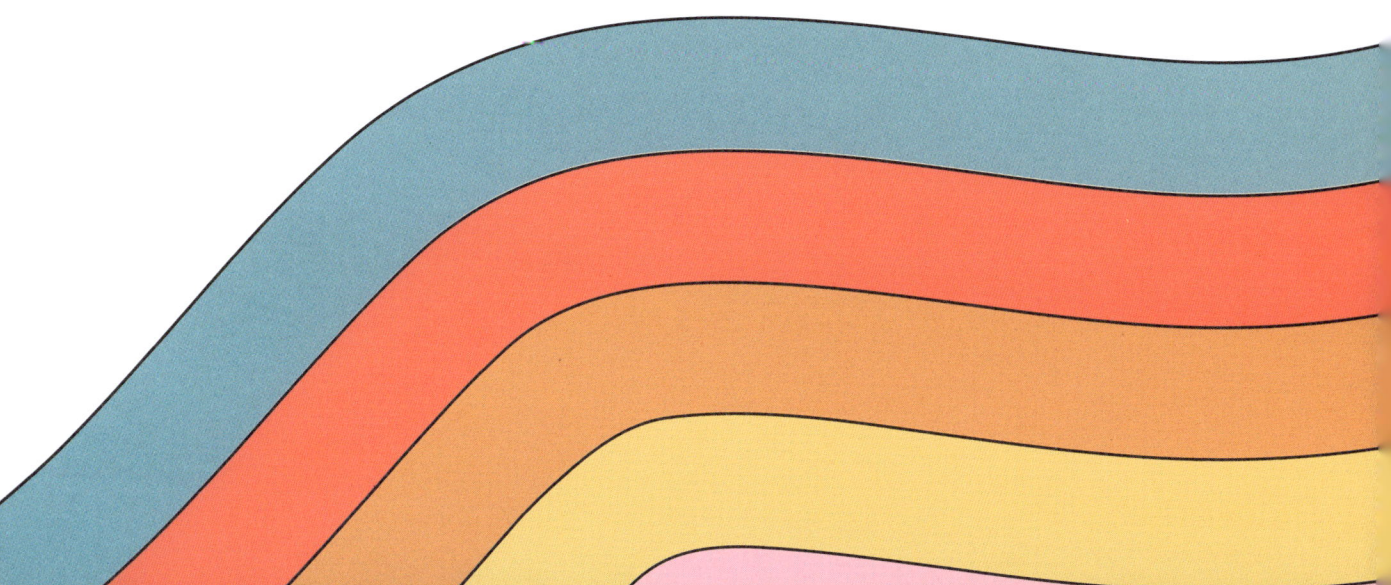

Take a second and stand or sit up tall like a tree with me.

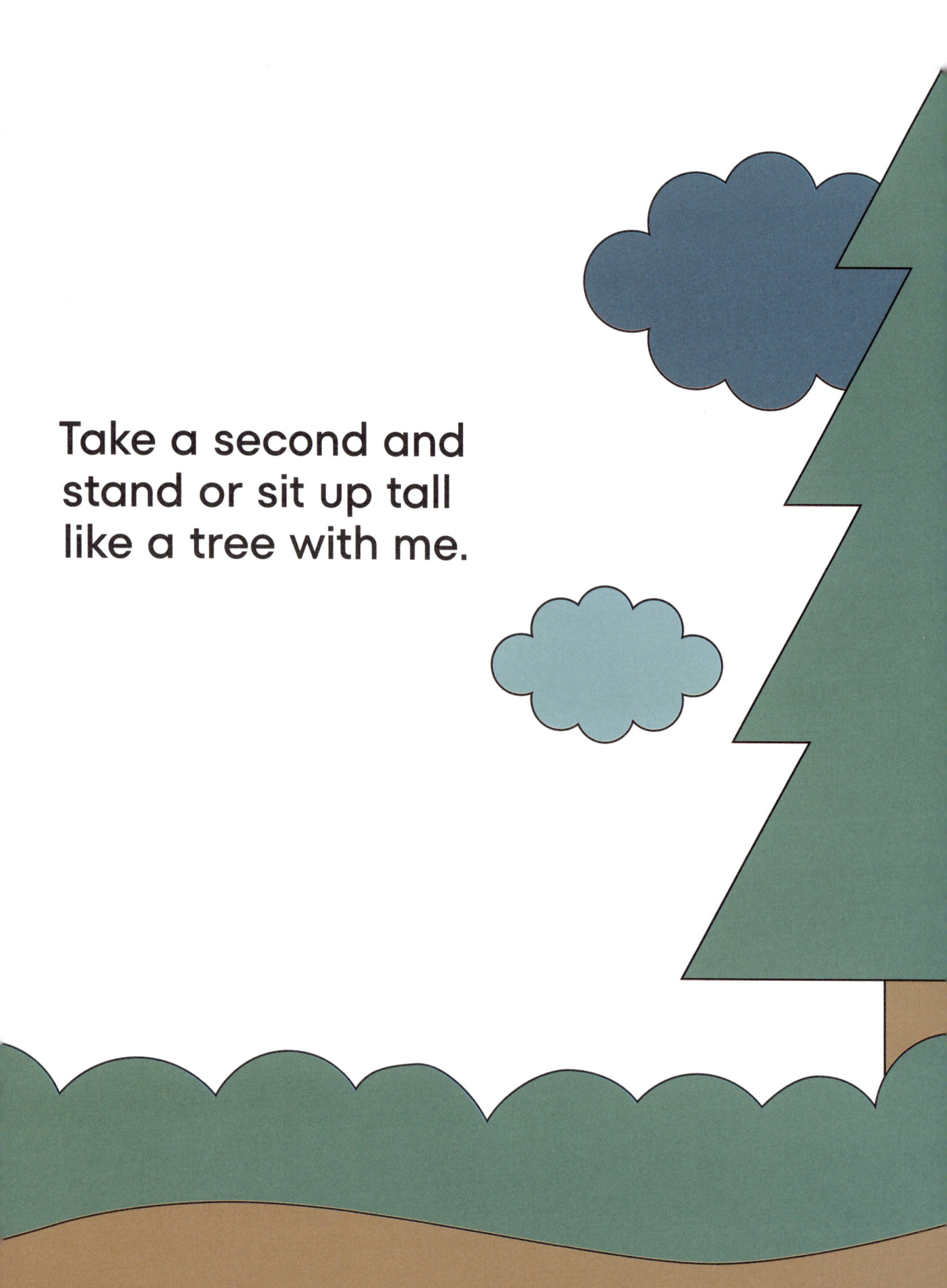

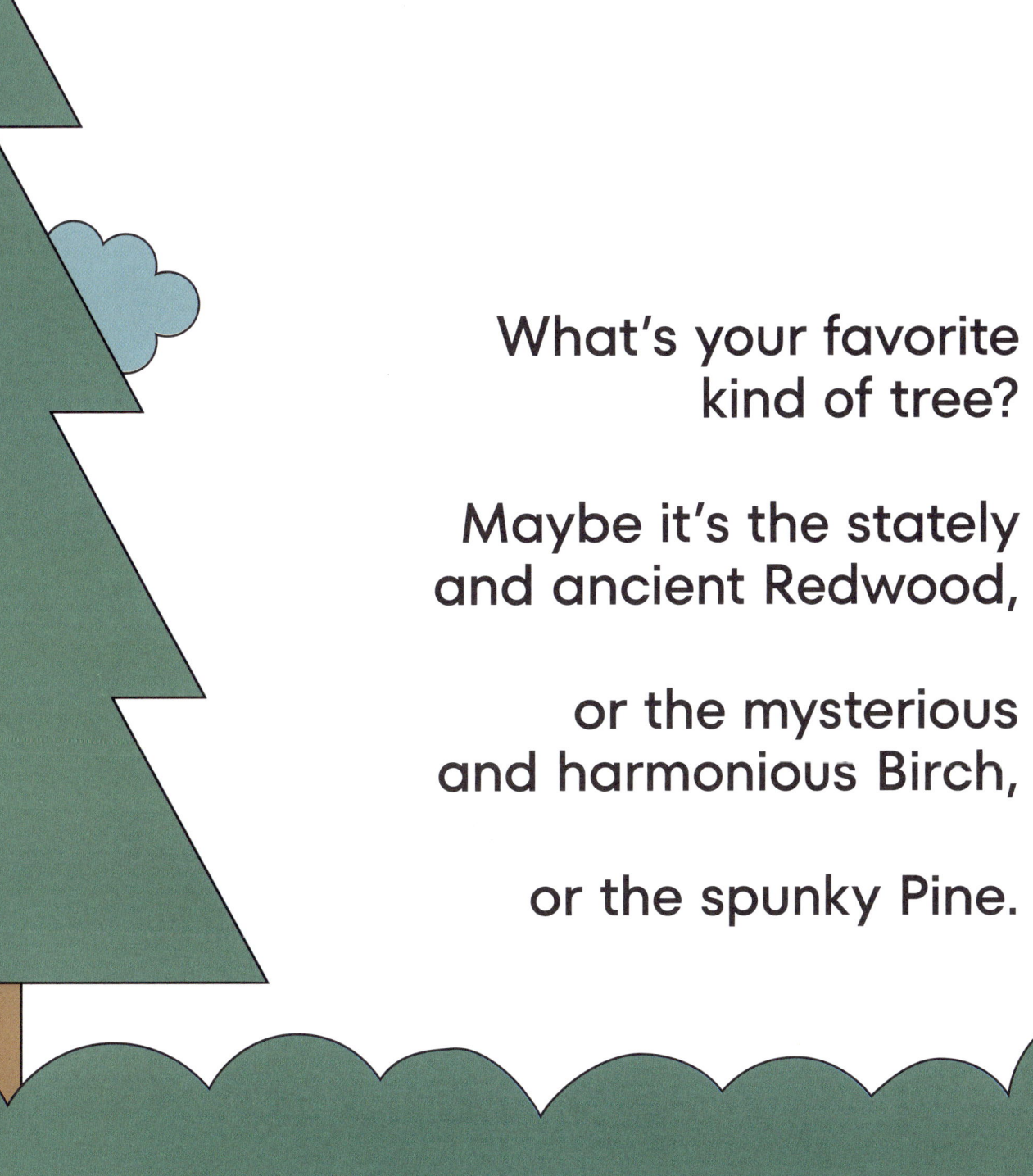

What's your favorite
kind of tree?

Maybe it's the stately
and ancient Redwood,

or the mysterious
and harmonious Birch,

or the spunky Pine.

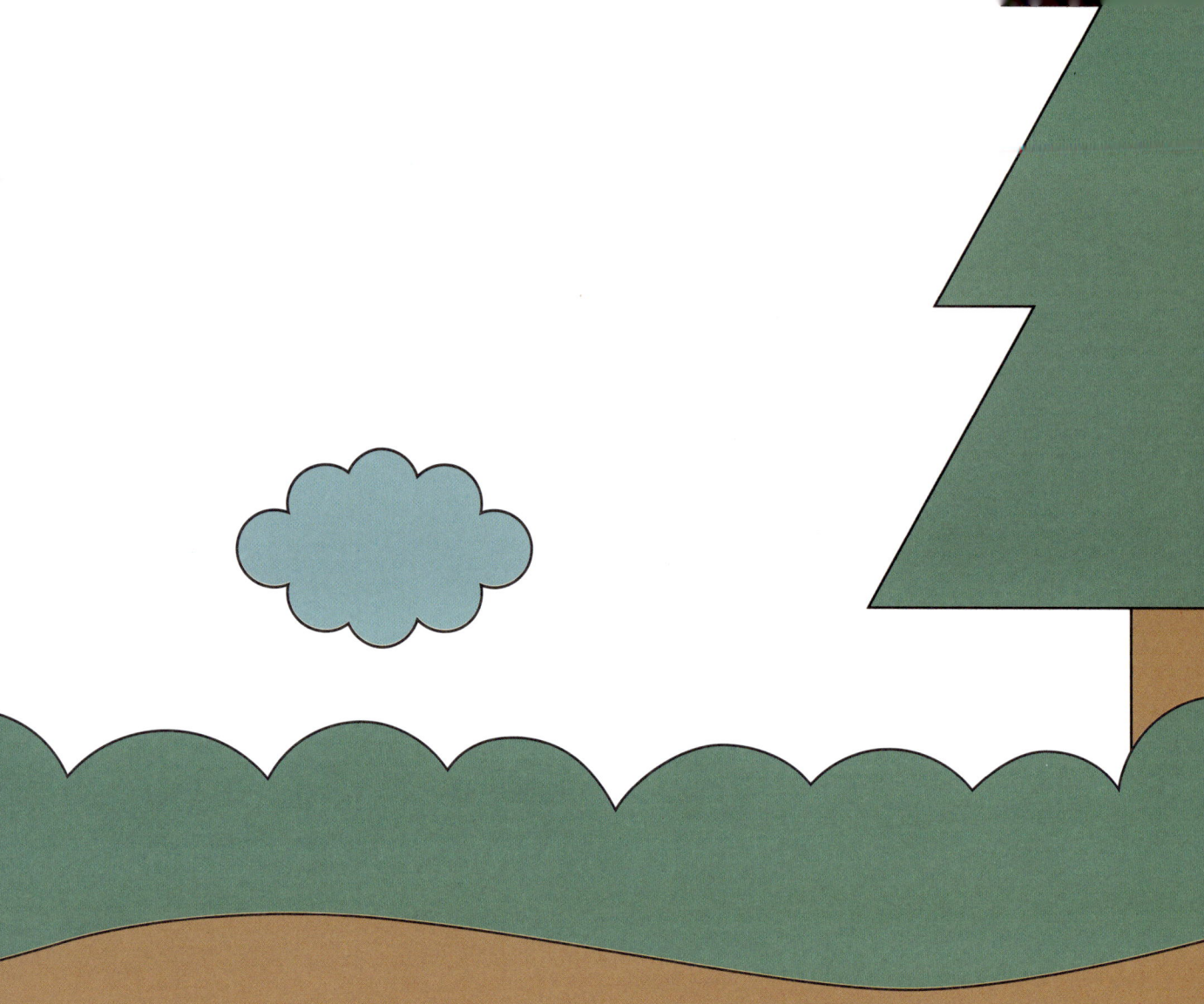

Imagine that roots are growing from your feet, deep into the soil.

Now, pretend to be the tree trunk: your legs, hips, mid-body, shoulders, and chest are strong and growing toward the sky.

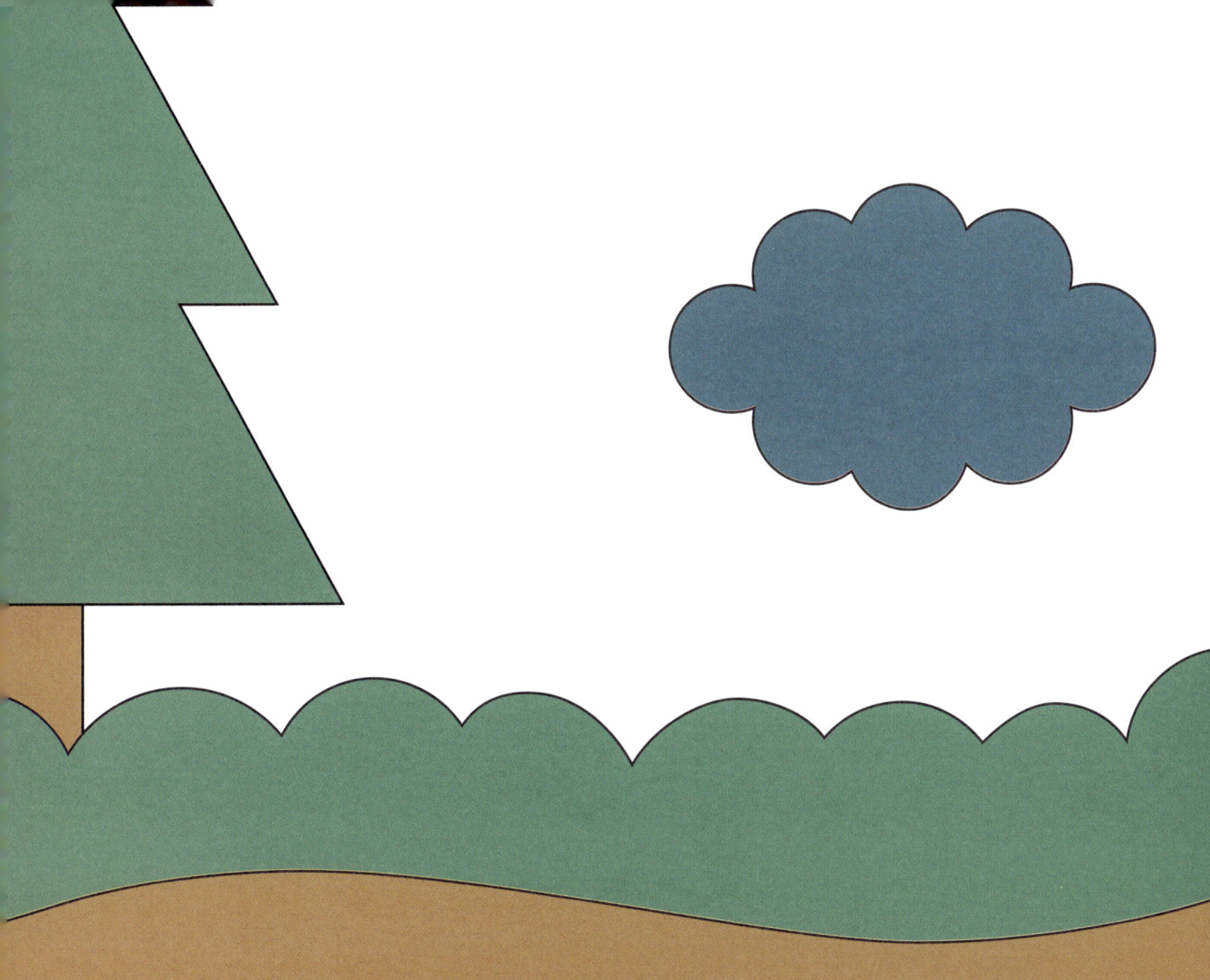

Ever so slowly, grow your branches up to the sky, turning your face upward like an opening leaf, ready to absorb the energy of the sun.

You are a majestic tree, strong and purposeful, part of the ecosystem surrounding you.

And even though
trees will always change...

from green leaves in springtime,

to burning fall colors,

to bare branches in the winter,

and the width of its trunk
growing each year...

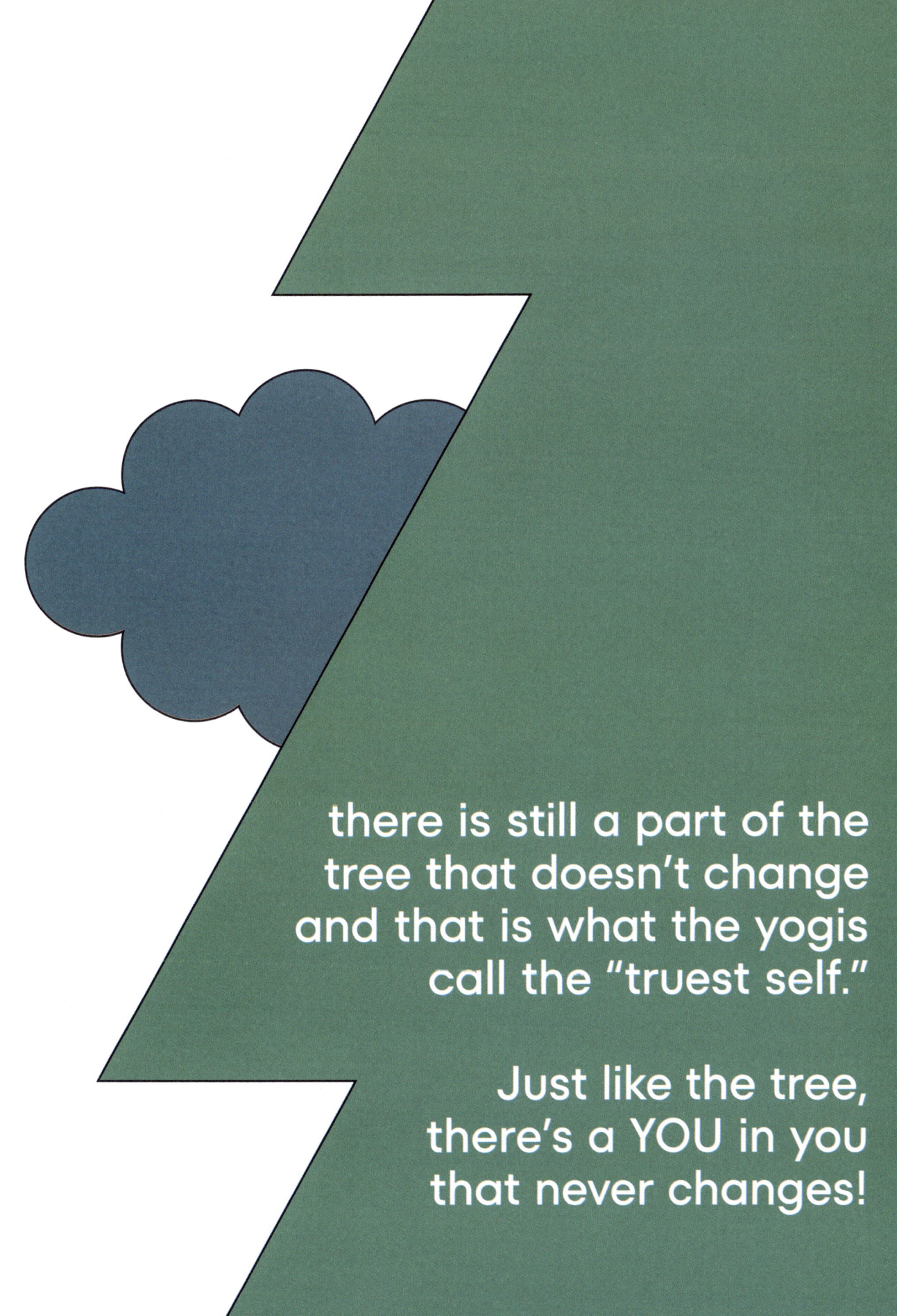

there is still a part of the tree that doesn't change and that is what the yogis call the "truest self."

Just like the tree, there's a YOU in you that never changes!

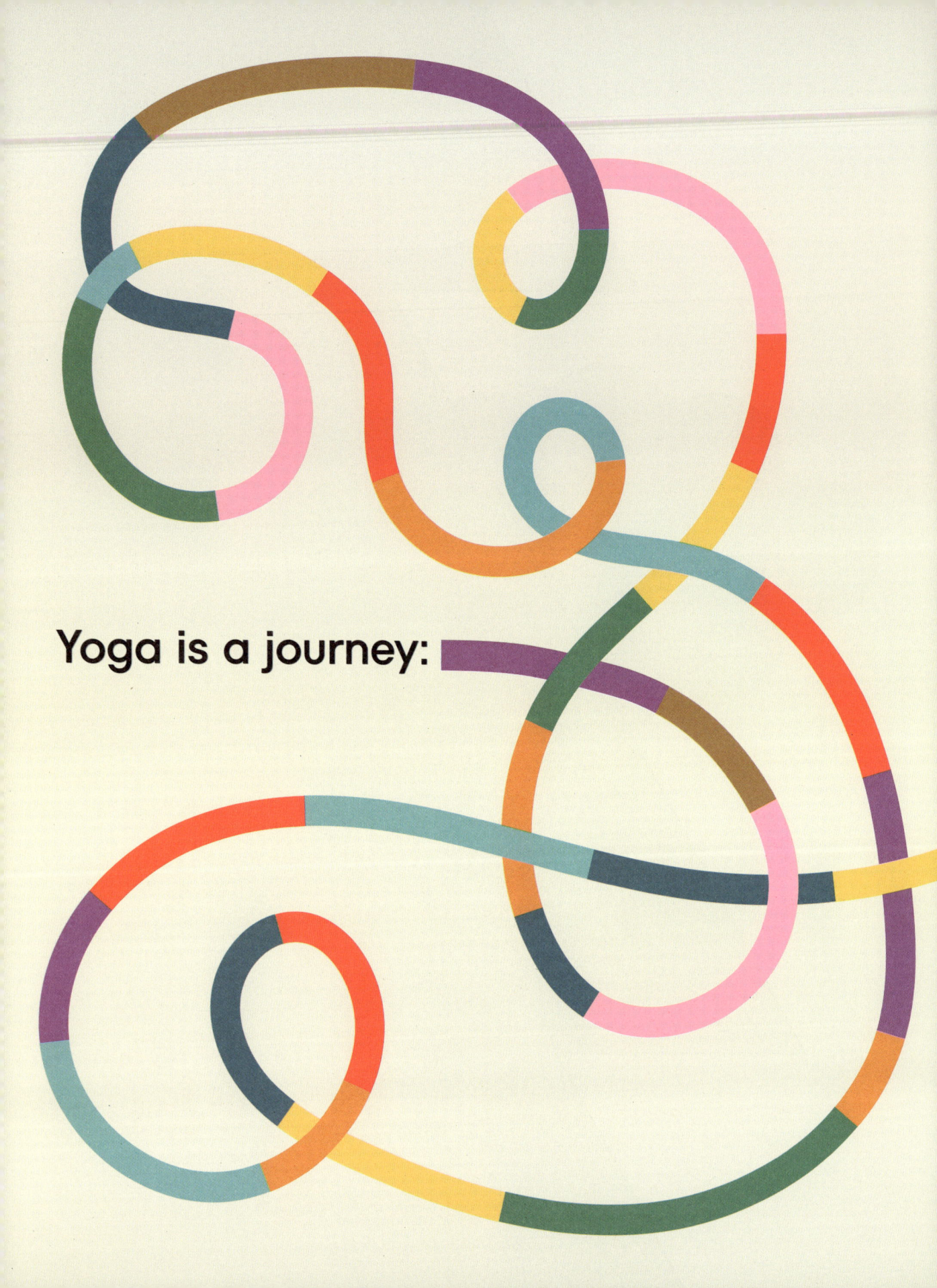

Yoga is a journey:

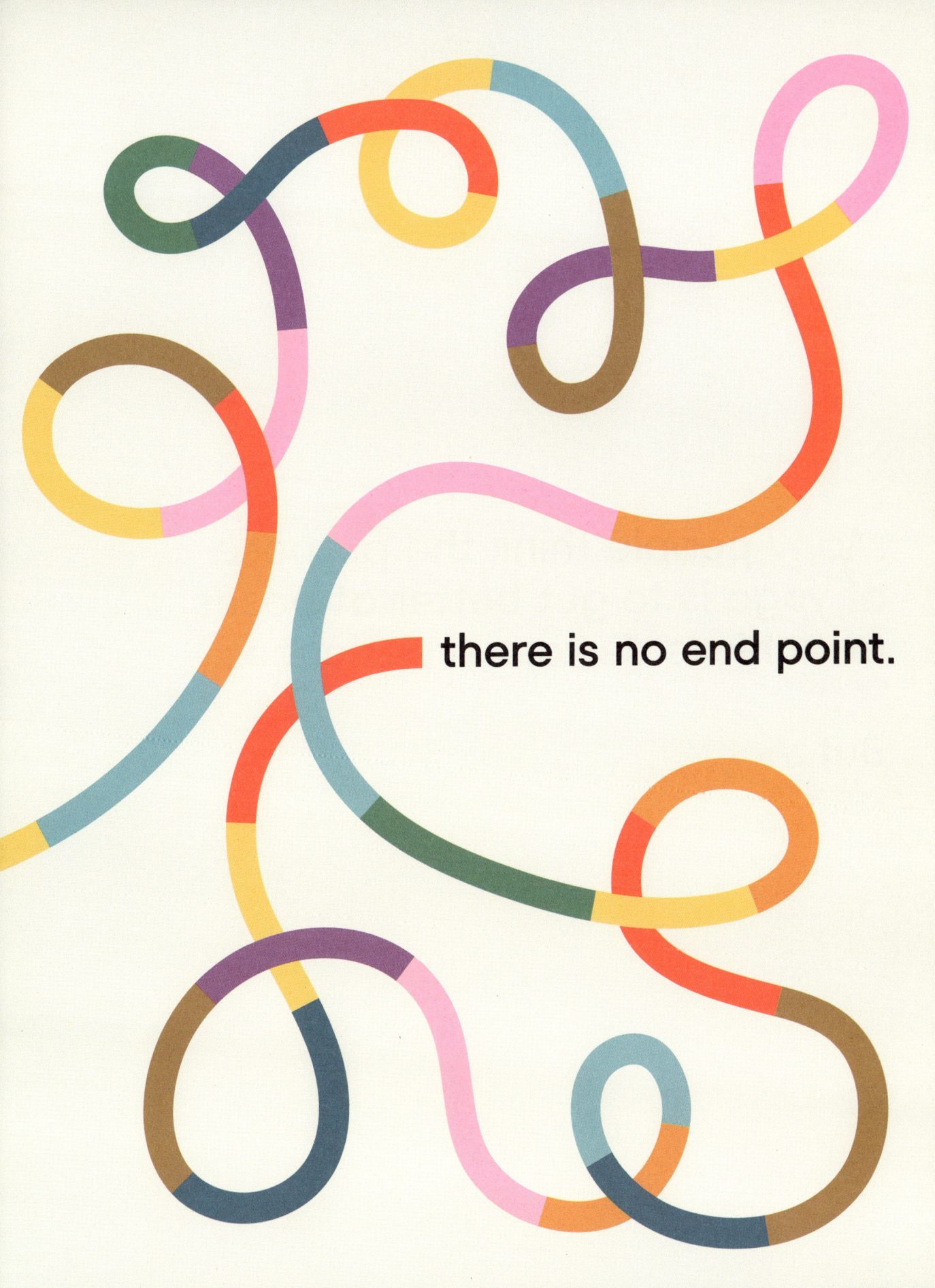

there is no end point.

Many people think the purpose of yoga is to get better at poses, or achieve certain experiences.

But...

# YOGA IS A JOURNEY BACK TO YOUR WHOLE SELF

(which has always been there, waiting for you to find it!).

It doesn't matter what you look like, or what doing yoga looks like to you.

Maybe it's sitting.

Maybe it's walking.

Maybe it's breathing.

Maybe it's doing poses.

Maybe it's loving your family or your community.

Maybe it's fighting for justice.

For many, it's a combination of these.

When I first started yoga, it was about me, how I wanted to feel in my body, and how I wanted to experience the world.

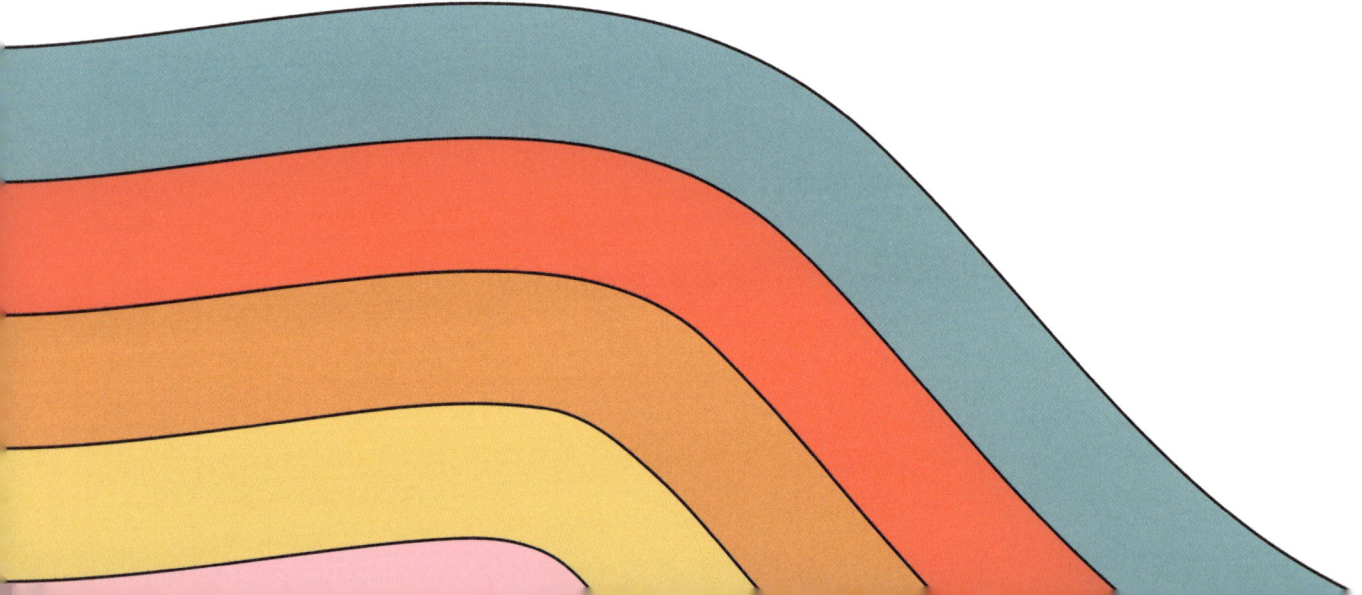

But now, I know it's about...

BEING MY TRUEST SELF, SO THOSE AROUND ME CAN DO THE SAME.

It's about doing my part to be free, so those around me can be free, and maybe one day, the whole world will be free, too.

# Outro
# for grownups

**N**ow that you've learned more about yoga, where can you go from here? You are already doing yoga a little bit each day, just by existing! Slowly, over time, you can build a stronger awareness of yoga's power in your life and tap into it when you need it!

Consider these questions with the kid(s) in your life:

Since yoga isn't just about doing poses, how are you doing yoga in your everyday life?

Where is one place where you feel like you can truly be yourself?

What does the most free, natural version of yourself look like? Feel like? Think about?

What are things you want to bring back together that were never meant to be apart?

Grownup, it's important to return to a free, natural state yourself—like when you were a kid. Remember what you loved, and use that as a guide. When you reconnect with your deepest self, your kid will begin to understand that they can do the same.

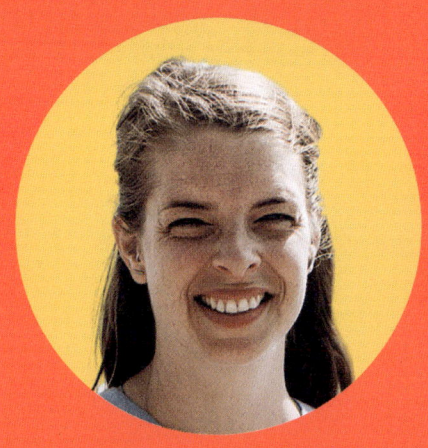

# About The Author

Megan Snider (she/her) wrote this book because she knew there was more than the surface-level interpretations of yoga she saw around her. Megan's journey with yoga for kids began when, on the last weekend of her yoga teacher training, she found out she was pregnant after years of infertility. She was in love with yoga and her baby, and she didn't want the 2 things to be separate. So, she started Appleseed Yoga—teaching kids yoga in schools and running a justice-focused kids yoga teacher training.

Megan wants to share the truth of yoga with the next generation so they can grow up with clearer, stronger senses of themselves. She deeply believes that as we navigate the distraction and confusion of life, if we can remember to return to the truth of ourselves, we can live with greater ease and love.

 @appleseedyoga

# Made to empower.

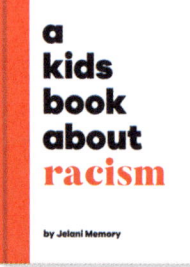
a kids book about racism
by Jelani Memory

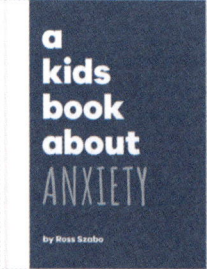
a kids book about ANXIETY
by Ross Szabo

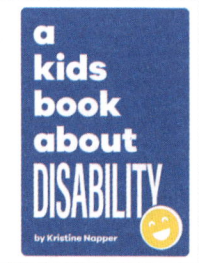
a kids book about DISABILITY
by Kristine Napper

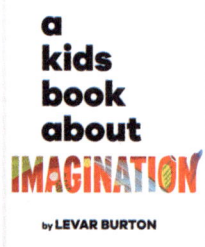
a kids book about IMAGINATION
by LEVAR BURTON

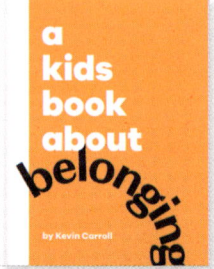
a kids book about belonging
by Kevin Carroll

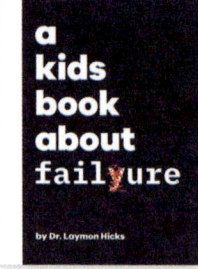
a kids book about failyure
by Dr. Laymon Hicks

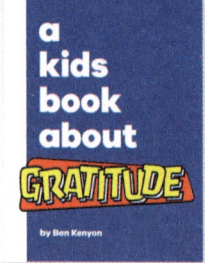
a kids book about GRATITUDE
by Ben Kenyon

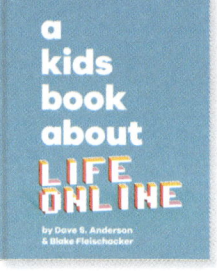
a kids book about LIFE ONLINE
by Dave S. Anderson & Blake Fleischacker

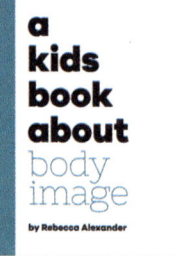
a kids book about body image
by Rebecca Alexander

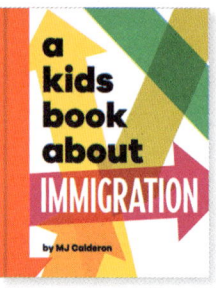
a kids book about IMMIGRATION
by MJ Calderon

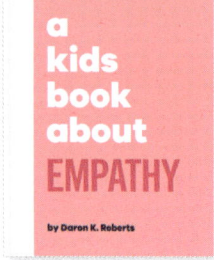
a kids book about EMPATHY
by Daron K. Roberts

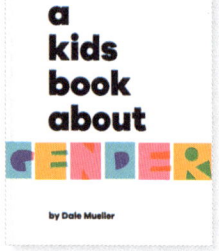
a kids book about GENDER
by Dale Mueller

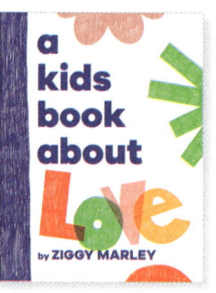
a kids book about Love
by ZIGGY MARLEY

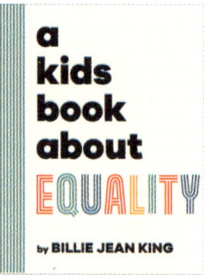
a kids book about EQUALITY
by BILLIE JEAN KING

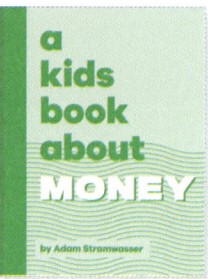
a kids book about MONEY
by Adam Stramwasser

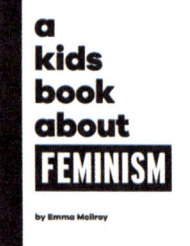
a kids book about FEMINISM
by Emma Mcilroy

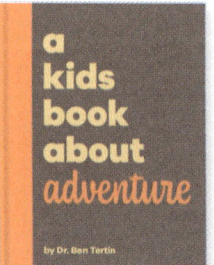
a kids book about adventure
by Dr. Ben Tertin

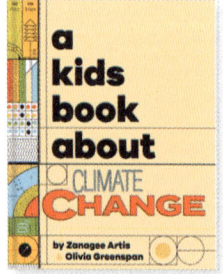
a kids book about CLIMATE CHANGE
by Zanagee Artis Olivia Greenspan

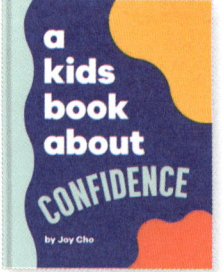
a kids book about CONFIDENCE
by Joy Cho

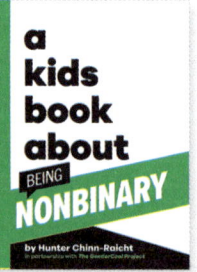
a kids book about BEING NONBINARY
by Hunter Chinn-Raicht
in partnership with The GenderCool Project

## Discover more at akidsco.com